Teachers of Healing and Wholeness

Huang Di

Also in this series

1 · ANDREW BOORDE: HEALING THROUGH MIRTH

2 · HIPPOCRATES: THE NATURAL REGIMEN

4 · PATANJALI: THE THREADS OF YOGA

Other titles in preparation

Teachers of Healing and Wholeness

Huang Di

The Balance of Yin and Yang

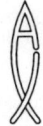

ARTHUR JAMES
BERKHAMSTED

First published in Great Britain by
ARTHUR JAMES LTD
70 Cross Oak Road
Berkhamsted
Hertfordshire HP4 3HZ

Introduction and selection:
© Robert Van de Weyer 1997

All rights reserved. No part of this book may be reproduced,
stored in a retrieval system, or transmitted by any means,
electronic, mechanical, photocopying, recording, or otherwise,
without the prior written permission of the publishers.

This book is sold subject to the condition that it shall not,
by way of trade or otherwise, be lent, re-sold, hired out
or otherwise circulated without the publisher's prior consent
in any form of binding or cover other than that in which
it is published and without a similar condition including
this condition being imposed on the subsequent purchaser.

A catalogue record for this book is available from
the British Library.

ISBN 0 85305 412 6

Typeset in Monotype Columbus by
Strathmore Publishing Services, London N7

Printed in Great Britain at
Ipswich Book Company, Ipswich, Suffolk

Contents

	Series Introduction	vii
	Introduction	ix
1	Wisdom and Folly	1
2	Yin and Yang	8
3	Body and Mind	12
4	Times and Seasons	19
5	Food and Air	24
6	Pulse and Complexion	31
7	Acupuncture and Moxa	37
8	Passion and Restraint	42

Series Introduction

At a time when the limitations of modern medicine are becoming clear, growing numbers of people are looking back to older approaches to healing and wholeness. The series aims to make available to the general reader original writings of the great teachers, from every part of the world and from every period of history.

The particular insights of the different teachers vary, and each has special wisdom for us to hear. Yet various themes recur. They all stress the unity of the spiritual and physical aspects of human nature, and therefore the need to care for the whole person. They emphasise the importance of the way we conduct our daily lives, both to prevent and to cure illness. And they seek to harness the latent powers of self-healing.

None of the healers in this series claimed to be infallible; all saw themselves as explorers. Thus none asked for uncritical trust; they regarded themselves as partners with those who listened to their words. In reading their works today we should see ourselves as partners, reflecting on what they say, and taking such advice as we think is right.

Introduction

Huang Di's *Book of Internal Medicine* is probably the oldest book on healing which we still possess; parts of it may have been composed over four thousand years ago. It contains the earliest exposition of the art of acupuncture, the most famous of Chinese healing techniques. Huang Di was also the first to apply the principle of Tao, and of Yin and Yang, to human health. Thus without doubt his work is of huge historical importance; and today it challenges western readers to look at themselves, and their own physical and mental needs and problems, with fresh eyes.

Huang Di, the 'Yellow Emperor', is supposed to have lived around 2600 BC. According to legend, he was a man of great ingenuity, inventing the wheel, the ship, and soldiers' armour. And during his reign the giraffe is said to have appeared in China, as a sign of his great wisdom. Since there are no documents or archaeological remains testifying to his various activities, some modern historians question his existence. There is no doubt. however, that from ancient times his name was associated with the classic work on Chinese medicine, and also with a parallel book on sexuality. These books had to be learnt by heart by all who wanted to work as healers and counsellors, and in this way they passed from one generation to the next. There is some evidence that they were written down around 1000 BC, and certainly they enjoyed wide circulation during the Ha Dynasty in the first century BC.

The word 'Tao' (pronounced 'Dow'), as expounded by Huang Di, has no direct English equivalent, since it embraces at least two western concepts. Firstly Tao is the divine spirit which infuses and permeates everything which exists; and secondly it is the way of life which obeys and conforms to this spirit. The terms 'Yin' and 'Yang' are equally elusive. Huang Di often refers to them as the female and male principles in nature, sometimes as Heaven and Earth. At various points in his book almost every polarity imaginable is encompassed in these two notions. Yang stands for sun, day, fire, heat, dryness and light; Yin for moon, night, water, cold, dampness and dark. Yang tends to expand, and to flow upwards and outwards; Yin to contract, and to flow downwards. Yang represents the sun and rain fertilising Yin, the soil. Yang signifies motion and activity; Yin signifies stillness and passivity. In terms of human temperament, Yang represents exuberance and joy while Yin represents melancholy and sadness.

In Huang Di's eyes, to obey Tao consists in

harmonising Yin and Yang in the conduct of one's life; this in turn will ensure good health and longevity. The early chapters of his book are largely devoted to instilling a healthy and harmonious way of life, and to describing the kinds of behaviour that will lead to disharmony between Yin and Yang, and thence to illness. This leads on to a more detailed exposition of how the body and the mind work, how they respond to the changing seasons, and how they are affected by the food consumed and the air breathed. Diagnosis of particular illness depends crucially on the pulse and the complexion, and Huang Di gives a detailed account of how the pulse should be taken and the complexion read so as to give maximum insight.

Generally, according to Huang Di, illnesses will be cured if the sick person leads a harmonious and balanced life, following the Tao. But the transition from sickness to health can be helped by acupuncture and moxa. As is now well-known in the west, acupuncture involves inserting needles into the body. Huang Di sees the purpose of acupuncture as draining away Yin or Yang where they are excessive, and replenishing them where they are lacking. He recounts how needles inserted in one place, such as the foot or hand, can affect organs elsewhere, such as the stomach or kidneys; however, in the book as we now possess it, there is no detailed analysis of these connection or 'meridians', nor a description of precisely where the needles should be put; we can assume that, like any craft, the techniques were passed on from one practitioner to another. Moxa has a similar purpose to acupuncture, and is applied to the same places, but does not use needles. Instead, the herb mugwort is ground into a powder, pressed into a ball, and placed on the patient's skin; the ball is then ignited, usually raising a blister.

Of all human activities, Huang Di regards sex as the most important. Sexual intercourse, he teaches, can be the supreme moment of unity between Yin and Yang, and thus bring greater physical and mental benefits. To achieve this unity men and women must harmonise their moods and emotions – for which he gives instructions. The most striking aspect of his sexual views is that the man should usually restrain his urge to ejaculate, and thus retain his semen. This, according to Huang Di, is physically beneficial, and also sustains his desire for the woman. More particularly it leads to a fuller unity of Yin and Yang, because the man and the woman will reach their climax in a more similar fashion.

In the form in which they come down to us, Huang Di's books are not easy to read and absorb – at least for the western mind. There is no clear structure or line of argument, and key ideas are frequently repeated in different contexts. Like many later Taoist writers,

INTRODUCTION

Huang Di is fascinated by numerical schemes, and his at-tempts to press his radical ideas into various numerical formulae often seem awkward and contrived. For these reasons, despite the huge growth of interest in ancient Chinese methods of healing, this classic work is virtually unread in the west. Yet Huang Di's Taoist philosophy, in its pure and ancient form, yields profound insights into human health, as well as priceless practical wisdom. He demonstrates, as clearly as any writer, how religion and healing are – or should be – one and the same.

I
Wisdom and folly

Temperance in All Things

In ancient times people understood Tao, and they ordered their lives according to the principles of Yin and Yang. Thus they were healthy; and most survived until they were over a hundred years of age, remaining fit and active to the day they died.

They were temperate in their eating and drinking. They were regular in their habits, rising and retiring at the same time each morning and evening. In this way they kept their bodies united with their souls, and so completed their allotted span.

Nowadays people are not like this. They drink wine to quench their thirst. They have no routine. They indulge their sexual appetites when they are intoxicated, and so exhaust themselves. They have no control over their emotions, and so do not know how to be peaceful and tranquil within themselves. They want only to amuse themselves, so they cut themselves off from the source of true joy. They rise and retire at different times each day. Thus they are mostly dead by the age of fifty, and long before death their bodies are beset by illness.

In ancient times people followed the teachings of the sages. These sages were serene and tranquil within themselves. They wanted nothing, and so were content with everything. They did not exhaust themselves, but preserved their life force. So how could illness overcome them?

They controlled their emotions, and minimised their desires. Their hearts were at peace, and free from fear. They toiled in the fields, but did not become weary.

They lived in harmony with their surroundings. They enjoyed the food that was right to eat. They took pleasure in wearing simple clothes. They never complained. They were indifferent to people's status, but treated everyone with equal kindness. They were pure in heart, so they could not be tempted by evil or excess.

– Book 1.1

Natural Living

Originally human beings lived amongst the birds and animals and reptiles. Like all other creatures, humans worked hard to find food during the day, and rested at night. There were no extended family ties, catching people in a web of duties and obligations, and there were no government officials imposing rules. Into this natural and free existence evil influences could not penetrate. So artificial treatments for illness, such as acupuncture and medicine, were not needed. When illness struck, it was sufficient simply to pray for healing.

But the present world is very different. People no longer live like other creatures, obeying the laws of nature; instead they rebel against these laws. Thus evil influences can penetrate at any time. These may injure the internal organs, or may damage the muscles and flesh. They may also enter the mind, causing anger, grief and confusion. Minor illnesses are apt to become serious; and serious illnesses often cause death. It is no longer sufficient to pray for healing.

– Book 4.2.

The Way of Contentment

Those who are wise control their desires, so that they want only what is good for them. In their hearts there is neither hatred nor anger. They do not try to separate themselves from the activities of the world, yet they are not slaves to custom. They work, but they do not over-exert their bodies. They meditate, but they do not over-exert their minds. Contentment is to them the highest achievement. Thus their bodies cannot be harmed, and their mental faculties cannot be dissipated.

– *Book 1.1*

Seeking the Truth

Those whose minds and spirits are constantly searching for truth will retain clear sight and sharp hearing; their bodies will remain light and strong, and although they grow old in years they will retain the physical abilities of youth. For this reason those who are wise do not concern themselves unduly with worldly affairs, nor do they indulge in extreme pleasures, because these things distract the mind and spirit from their true purpose. They devote themselves to contemplation and to study, and they find pleasure in quietness and tranquillity.

– *Book 2.1*

True Desires

Wise people who are aware of the true needs and desires of the body, and who satisfy those needs and desires, remain healthy; and good health helps them to become peace-loving and virtuous. Foolish people who ignore the needs and desires of the body are prone to illness; their bodies are constantly tense and nervous, so they are quick to become angry and unkind.

– *Book 3.1*

The Consequences of Excess (1)

Excess of anything – food, sex, emotion, exercise, rest, drink – causes unbalance and disharmony in the body, mind and spirit.

Excess causes a person to forget what is right and good, and to become morally lax.

Excess causes a person's body to become hot, and the skin and flesh to ache.

Excess causes a person to produce too much phlegm and saliva, which induces coughing and spitting.

Excess causes a person to pant, and to have difficulty breathing.

Excess weakens a person, making the back prone to injury and pain.

Excess causes a person to slump, rather than sit upright, which eventually induces chronic pain.

Excess causes a person to feel anxious, even when there is no outside reason.

Excess causes a person to become stiff in the limbs, so that eventually the limbs can barely move.

– *Book 4.7*

The Consequences of Excess (2)

Those who do not breathe deeply and steadily find that evil influences enter the body, and the liver is injured. Those who overeat find that the pulse weakens, the muscles collapse, and the bowels are injured, causing piles which bleed. Those who drink in excess become angry and obstreperous. Those who have sexual intercourse too frequently injure the kidneys, and strain the loins.

— Book 1.3

Attention to Oneself

Those who wish to be healthy should first give attention to the skin, ensuring the complexion is clear, and to the hair, ensuring it is clean and shiny. They should then give attention to the muscles, ensuring through appropriate exercise that these remain strong and supple, and to the flesh, ensuring that the body becomes neither too fat nor too thin. They should then give attention to the bowels, ensuring through diet and exercise that there is neither constipation nor diarrhoea. Finally they should give attention to the internal organs.

— Book 2.1

Obeying Nature

Those who are wise obey the laws of nature. So their bodies are free from strange diseases, and they do not lose the faculties with which Nature has endowed them. Their vital spirit is never exhausted.

— *Book 1.2*

Preserving Vitality

Foolish people wear out their bodies and exhaust their blood; and they wear out their minds and exhaust their spirits. When this has happened, no treatment can restore their vitality. Wise people live in such a way that their vitality is preserved, and their energy is constantly replenished. The healer should be bold enough to criticise those whose way of life is exhausting them and wearing them out.

— *Book 4.2*

Purity

Just as the breath of blue sky is calm, so the will and the heart of those who are pure is calm. — *Book 1.3*

2
Yin and Yang
• • • • • • • • • • • • •

The Universal Principle (1)

The principle of Yin and Yang is the basic principle of the entire universe. It is the root and source of life and death. In order to treat and cure diseases one must understand this principle.

Heaven was created by an accumulation of Yang, the essence of light. Earth was created by an accumulation of Yin, the essence of darkness.

— *Book 2.3*

The Universal Principle (2)

Obedience to the laws of Yin and Yang means life; disobedience means death. Obedience brings harmony and order; disobedience brings confusion and disorder.

— *Book 1.2*

Different Faculties

Yang is the element of light. The essences of Yang unite and ascend to Heaven, creating clarity and light above. Yin is the element of darkness. The essences of Yin unite and descend to Earth, creating fullness and abundance below. Yin enables people to use their hands and feet well.

— *Book 2.1*

Unified Spirit

If Yin and Yang do not harmonise and unite, it is like spring without autumn, or winter without summer. The life force is destroyed. But if Yin is in a state of tranquillity, and Yang is strong, then the spirit is content.

— *Book 1.3*

Signs of Imbalance

Yin is active within the body, and regulates Yang. Yang is active on the outside of the body, and regulates Yin. When Yang is too strong, the body becomes hot, and the person starts to pant; the mouth becomes dry, and the bowels become constipated. For a person in such a condition the heat of summer is unendurable. When Yin is too strong, the body becomes cold, and the limbs start to tremble; the stomach cannot digest food properly, so the person suffers diarrhoea. For a person in such a condition the cold of winter is unendurable.

– Book 2.1

Preserving Balance

Yin stores up the essences within the body, and prepares them for use. Yang uses those essences, protecting the body from external danger. If Yin is less than Yang, the pulse becomes weak, the body sickly, and the mind confused. If Yang is less than Yin, the internal organs conflict with one another, and the orifices become blocked. Thus those who are wise keep Yin and Yang in balance. They eat appropriately to ensure the pulse and the muscles are in harmony; they exercise in order to make their bones and marrow strong; they breathe deeply and steadily. By keeping Yin and Yang in balance the eyes remain clear, the ears remain alert, and the mind remains sharp. Thus the life force is kept in its original, pristine state.

– Book 1.2

YIN AND YANG

Different Characters

Those who are peaceful and quiet are influenced by Yin; those who are active are influenced by Yang. Those who are slow and dilatory are influenced by Yin; those who are quick are influenced by Yang. Those influenced by Yin are more prone to diseases of the internal organs. Those influenced by Yang are prone to diseases of the external organs.

– Book 2.3

Stress

When a person too frequently becomes angry or frightened, the force of Yang overwhelms Yin. Ulcers appear on the skin and on the internal organs. The orifices, especially the nose and throat, are liable to become blocked. The person can also suffer flatulence and intermittent fevers, and the complexion becomes red.

The wise person learns to prevent this happening. But if it does occur, the person should try to dissipate the excess Yang through rest and relaxation. Acupuncture may assist in removing blockages which have formed, allowing the excess Yang to drain away.

– Book 1.3

HUANG DI

Wanting Wholeness

The wise healer does not attempt to treat those who are ill yet who have no wish to obey the laws of Yin and Yang. The wise healer treats those who are well and who want to avoid illness, and those who are ill and want to reform their lives according to the laws of Yin and Yang.

— *Book 1.2*

3
Body and Mind

Internal and External Organs

The organs of the human body which relate to the outside world are Yang; the internal organs are Yin. There are five internal organs belonging to Yin: liver, heart, pancreas, lungs and kidneys. There are five external organs belonging to Yang: gall-bladder, stomach, intestines, urinary bladder and the triple heater [the meaning of this is uncertain – Ed.]. – *Book 1.4*

Functions and Signs of Internal Organs

The heart is the root of life, and thus controls the spiritual faculties. It fills the pulse with blood, and influences the face. The complexion of a person reveals the condition of the heart.

The lungs are the origin of breath, and are where the animal spirit of a person is located. They are connected with the skin and the hair. The sheen of a person's hair reveals the condition of the lungs.

The liver is the source of energy, and is where the soul which ascends to Heaven lives. It is connected with the muscles, and the nails. The state of a person's finger and toe nails, and the amount of energy a person has, reveal the condition of the liver.

The kidneys are where the vital essences are stored. They are connected with the bones. The strength and hardness of a person's bones reveal the condition of the kidneys.

The pancreas is the source of transformation, enabling a person to change from good to evil, or evil to good. The stomach is connected with the flesh. The colour of a person's lips reveals the condition of the stomach.

— *Book 3.1 and 3.2*

The Body as a Kingdom

The heart is like the minister to a monarch, who offers the monarch insight and wisdom. The lungs are the rules which inspire and guide the conduct of all the monarch's officials. The liver is like the military leader who excels in strategic planning The gall bladder is an important and upright official on whom the monarch can rely for sound judgement. The triple heater is the official who arranges dramas and pageants, to give pleasure to the monarch's subjects. The stomach is the official that looks after the public granaries. The intestine is the moral guide, who shows people the right way to live. The pancreas is the economic guide, who shows people how to work. The kidneys are the philosophers, who purify people's thoughts. The urinary bladder is the magistrate who takes away all that is impure. All these various people assist one another in a successful and prosperous kingdom; all the various organs must assist one another within a healthy and thriving person.

– Book 3.1

Head and Back

The head is the home of skill and intelligence. When the head is constantly bowed, so the person is only looking down, eventually the spirit will be broken. The back is the main wall of the home where all the internal organs reside. When the back is constantly bent, through carrying heavy burdens, the internal organs will be crushed.

– Book 4.5

Breath as Symptom

If the breath is too plentiful, this indicates that disease is likely to occur in the external organs. If breath is too little, this indicates that disease has reached the internal organs.

— *Book 6.1*

Emotional Imbalance

There are five emotions: joy, anger, sympathy, grief and fear. If one of these emotions becomes dominant, the spirit is injured, causing severe spiritual pain. This may in time injure the internal organs, causing physical illness.

Extreme joy may injure the heart. Extreme anger injures the liver. Extreme sympathy injures the pancreas. Extreme grief injures the lungs. Extreme fear injures the kidneys and bowels.

The antidote to joy is fear; to anger is sympathy; to sympathy is anger; to grief is joy; to fear is contemplation.

— *Book 2.1*

Self-expression

The healer should seek to open the mind and hearts of patients, and let them express their feelings. Those who can express interest in the people and things around them, and possess a sense of purpose, are likely to overcome their illness. Those who can find no interest in people and things, and have lost all sense of purpose, are likely to be overcome by their illness.

– *Book 4.2*

Dreams and Diagnosis

When Yin is excessive, and thus overwhelming Yang, the person will have terrifying dreams of wading or swimming, and almost drowning. When Yang is excessive, and thus overwhelming Yin, the person will have terrifying dreams of being caught in fires, and almost burning to death. When Yin and Yang are both strong, but in conflict, the person will have dreams of fighting and warfare.

When there is an excess of joy, the person will dream of flying. When there is an excess of grief, the person will dream of falling down. When there is an excess of anger, the person will dream of violence. When there is an excess of sympathy, the person will dream of gliding through water like a fish. When there is an excess of fear, the person will dream of having insects buzzing around.

Those who are eating too much dream of being slim and nimble. Those who are eating too little dream of wonderful meals.

— *Book 4.5*

4
Times and Seasons

Through the Day

At dawn the breath of Yang is activated; at midday the breath of Yang is at its most abundant; as the sun moves to the west, the breath of Yang declines; when the sun sets, the breath of Yang can again barely be discerned. The breath of Yang warms the flesh and loosens the muscles, enabling the muscles to work well. If the flesh is exposed to the cold mists and dews of the night, the muscles become rigid, and their strength is lost.

– *Book 1.3*

Spring

The three months of Spring are the period when life begins and is renewed. The breaths of Heaven and Earth give birth and restore energy to all things.

In Spring people should rise early. They should first have a brisk walk, and then a leisurely stroll.

During the Spring people should be gentle with

their bodies. They should give their bodies rewards, not punishments. They should learn to take pleasure in what Nature offers.

Those who defy the laws of Spring will suffer injury to the liver. And in Summer they will catch chills.

– Book 1.3

Summer

The three months of Summer are the period of luxuriant growth. The breaths of Heaven and Earth intermingle, making all things bloom.

In Summer people should rise early. In the heat of the day they should not weary themselves. They should not allow themselves to become angry.

During the Summer people should concentrate on developing the best features of both their minds and their bodies. Through breathing deeply, they should bring the outside world deep within their bodies. They should love every aspect of the outside world.

Those who defy the laws of Summer will suffer injury to the heart. And in the Autumn they will feel weak, unable to stand the colder weather.

– Book 1.2

Autumn

The three months of Autumn are the period of tranquillity. The atmosphere of Heaven is serene, and the atmosphere of Earth is clear.

In Autumn people should retire early at night, and rise in the morning with the crowing of the rooster. They should keep their minds peaceful.

During Autumn people should not give expression to their physical desires. They should turn inwards, and concentrate on their souls. They should beware of breathing air that is foul or impure.

Those who defy the laws of Autumn will suffer injury to the lungs. And in Winter they will be prone to indigestion and diarrhoea. *— Book 1.2*

Winter

The three months of Winter are the period of death in life. Water freezes and Earth cracks open; Heaven is dormant.

In Winter people should retire early at night, and rise late with the rising of the sun. They should try to escape the cold and seek warmth; yet from time to time they should breathe in the cold air.

During Winter people should suppress and conceal their desires, as if all their wishes had already been fulfilled. They should not try to achieve anything, freeing their hearts from any urge to assert their will.

Those who defy the laws of Winter will suffer injury to the kidneys and testicles. And in Spring they will be impotent.

— *Book 2.1*

Self-development through the Year

The interaction of the four seasons and the interaction of Yin and Yang is the foundation of everything in the world. Those who are wise nurture and develop their Yang in Spring and Summer, and nurture and develop their Yin in Autumn and Spring. Those who fail to do this sever their own roots, causing themselves to wither and die.

— *Book 1.2*

Injuries through the Year

Those who are injured in the summer by heat will suffer intermittent fever in the autumn. Those who are injured in the autumn through humidity will suffer cough and impotence in the winter. Those who are injured in the winter through extreme cold will be weak and slow in the spring.

— *Book 1.2*

Fevers and Chills

Exposure of the body to extreme cold induces intense heat in the form of fevers. Exposure of the body to intense heat induces extreme cold in the form of chills.

— *Book 2.1.*

Heat Stroke

If people try to hurry in the heat of summer, or they become angry, they start to pant furiously, and sweat pours from them. And when they calm down, their minds are confused. Their bodies resemble burning charcoal. In this situation they must rest quietly, allowing the perspiration to carry away the fever. But if they persist in their folly, their Yang becomes exhausted, the orifices of the body become blocked, and they may even cease to sweat. They will then collapse, and it may be impossible to halt the onset of death.

— *Book 1.3*

5
Food and Air

Five Flavours

There are five flavours: sourness, saltiness, sweetness, bitterness and pungency. If sourness exceeds the other flavours, an excess of saliva and phlegm is produced, blocking the orifices. If saltiness exceeds the other flavours, the bones become weary, the heart becomes weak, and the mind anxious. If sweetness exceeds the other flavours, the lungs become breathless, the complexion darkens, and the kidneys become unbalanced. If bitterness exceeds the other flavours, the body becomes dry, and the stomach becomes heavy and upset. If pungency exceeds the other flavours, the muscles and the pulse become slack, and the mind depressed. It is important, therefore, to balance and mix the five flavours well. In this way the bones will remain straight, the muscles will remain tender, the breath will remain regular and deep, the blood will circulate freely, and the complexion will be clear.

— Book 1.3

Unbalanced Diet (1)

When flavours are unbalanced in the food we eat, and one strong flavour dominates, the Yin is weakened. This allows the Yang to dominate. The result is that passions become excessively strong, exhausting the body and confusing the mind. — *Book 2.1*

Unbalanced Diet (2)

If there is too much salt in food, the pulse hardens, eyes become watery, and the complexion becomes dull. If too much bitter flavour is used in food, the skin becomes withered and wrinkled, and hair loses its sheen. If too much pungent flavour is used, the muscles become knotted, and the finger and toe nails become brittle. If too much sour flavour is used, the flesh hardens and the lips become slack. If too much sweetness is used, the bones ache and become weary.

The heart craves bitter flavour, the lungs crave pungent flavour, the liver craves sour flavour, the stomach craves sweet flavour, the kidneys crave salt flavour. If the five flavours are correctly combined and balanced, all the internal organs will be satisfied and remain healthy.

— *Book 3.3*

Illnesses from Different Diets

The food which people eat, and their way of life, affects their state of health, and makes them prone to particular types of illness. Each type of illness has its own cure.

Those who live near the sea eat much fish and salt. Fish can cause internal burning, and excessive salt injures the blood. This diet can also cause ulcers. These illnesses are treated with acupuncture, using a needle made of flint.

Those who live on hills and mountains consume meat and milk. They wear rough woollen cloth. Their bodies are robust and strong. But the extreme cold may causes diseases of the their external bodies, in their muscles and skin. These are treated with moxibustion, cauterising with dried tinder.

Those who live in lush valleys eat much grain and vegetables. Such a health diet means that they rarely suffer diseases of their external bodies. But they also tend to be lazy and lax in their habits, and thus are prone to illness of the internal organs. These are treated with herbal medicines.

Those who live in dry areas drink little, and they crave sour foods such as curds. Their bones tend to bend, and their muscles contract and become numb.

These illnesses are treated with acupuncture, using fine metal needles.

Those who live in very wet areas, with dense woods, eat much fruit and nuts. They are prone to chills and fevers. These are treated with breathing exercises, with massage of the skin and flesh, and with exercises of the hands and feet.

– Book 4.1

Diets for Different Illnesses

Those with disease of the liver should eat only a little pungent food to prevent their liver from disintegrating, and sour food to drain the liver of excessive fullness.

Those with disease of the heart should only eat a little salty food to make the heart pliable, and then sweet foods such as fruits to drain the heart of excessive fullness.

Those with disease of the stomach should eat less than they desire. They should have only a little sweet food to set the stomach at ease, and then eat bitter food to drain the stomach of excessive fullness.

Those with disease of the lungs should eat sour food to strengthen the lungs, and then pungent food to drain the lungs of excessive fullness.

Those with disease of the kidneys should eat bitter

food to strengthen the kidneys, and then salty food to drain the kidneys of excessive fullness.

— *Book 7.2*

Mixing Herbs (1)

In herbs we taste all the five flavours: bitterness, sourness, sweetness, pungency and saltiness. The five flavours can be perfectly balanced and blended by mixing the herbs correctly. Then, when they are eaten and stored in the stomach, they will spread a health atmosphere through the body and the mind.

— *Book 3.1*

Mixing Herbs (2)

The most powerful parts of a herb in curing diseases are the extremities: the tips of the branches, and the tips of the roots. — *Book 4.2*

Soup for Illness (1)

When a disease of an internal organ begins, the person should consume only hot water and rice soup for ten

FOOD AND AIR

days. Only after this period, if the disease is not yet cured, should medicines be taken. Disease of the external organs do not require reduction in diet.

— *Book 4.2*

Soup for Illness (2)

To prepare soup for those who are sick the rice should be steamed, using the stalks of the rice as firewood. When the steaming is complete, the rice extract is very strong.

— *Book 4.2*

Illnesses from Different Weather (1)

The different winds may induce different illnesses. The wind blowing from the sea causes problems to the throat, nose and neck. The opposite wind blowing from the land causes problems to the shoulder and back. The warm south wind can cause disturbance to the chest and ribs. The cold north wind can cause problems in the loins and thighs. So, depending on which way the wind is blowing, people should be gentle towards the parts of the body which are most vulnerable.

— *Book 1.4*

Illnesses from Different Weather (2)

Oppressive humid weather upsets the mind, causing madness. Constant wind upsets the stomach, making it unable to retain food and digest it. Frosty air causes ulcers.

— *Book 5.1*

6
Pulse and Complexion

Observing Symptoms (1)

If you want to understand illness, observe yourself. Learn to notice small changes in yourself, and see from experience how these are symptoms of internal disturbance.

— *Book 2.1*

Observing Symptoms (2)

The good healer can discern disease before the person is aware of symptoms. This is done by sensing whether the body is in harmony with itself; if not, disease will ensue. The poor healer can only discern disease when the symptoms are already rampant.

— *Book 8.2*

Observing Symptoms (3)

The sages of old understood well that the complexion and the pulse are the two most valuable means of discerning a person's condition. The complexion corresponds with the sun; the pulse with the moon. Through experience and discernment the healer comes to understand their meaning. The complexion changes as the pulse changes; the one reflects the other.

– Book 4.2.

Taking the Pulse

The pulse should be taken at dawn when the breath of Yin has not yet begun to stir, and when the breath of Yang has not yet begun to diffuse; when food and drink have not yet been taken; and when energy has not yet been exerted. *– Book 4.5*

The Pulse through the Seasons

A healthy person has one exhalation of breath to two pulse beats, and one inhalation of breath to two pulse beats.

In Spring the pulse should be fine and delicate like the strings of a musical instrument.

In Summer the pulse should be like the beats of a fine hammer.

In the Autumn the pulse should be soft and gentle like a lullaby.

PUSLE AND COMPLEXION

In the Winter the pulse should be small and hard, like a stone. — *Book 4.6*

Interpreting the Pulse Beat

When the pulse beat is very deep and thin, this indicates excess Yin in the body. The person will tend to suffer chills.

When the pulse beat is hasty and panting, this indicates excess Yang in the body. The person will tend to suffer fevers. — *Book 4.5*

When the pulse beats are soft and scattered, yet the complexion is clear and shiny, this indicates the body is dehydrated; the person must drink more fluids.

— *Book 4.5*

When the pulse beats are very quick, so that there are six beats to every cycle of breath, this indicates disease of the heart.

When the pulse beat is very loud, this indicates disease of the pancreas. — *Book 4.5*

When the pulse is very full and slow, this indicates disease of the stomach, so the person is prone to indigestion. — *Book 5.1*

When the pulse is empty and slow, this indicates confusion of the brain.

When the pulse is full and quick, this indicates the person is prone to headaches.

When the pulse is large and heavy, this indicates disease of the kidneys.

– *Book 3.3.*

Interpreting the Complexion (1)

The healer should feel the person's pulse, and at the same time look deeply into the person's face to observe the complexion. In this way subtle colours in the complexion can be discerned.

If there is the colour red, this indicates evil influences in the heart. The diagnosis is confirmed if the person also suffers a persistent cough.

If there is the colour white, this indicates evil influence in the lungs. The diagnosis is confirmed if the person has a light cough and is short of breath. Evil influence in the lungs is associated with fevers and chills.

If there is the colour green, this indicates evil influence in the liver. The diagnosis is confirmed if there is lack of energy in the limbs, and if the feet hurt. Evil influence in the liver is associated with headaches.

If there is the colour yellow, this indicates evil influence in the pancreas. The diagnosis is confirmed if the person perspires excessively. Evil influence in the pancreas is associated with flatulence.

If there is the colour black, this indicates evil influence in the kidneys. The diagnosis is confirmed if the person is restless.

– *Book 3.3*

Interpreting the Complexion (2)

The healer may discern diseases of other organs of the body by looking at a person's complexion, observing subtle colours beneath the surface.

If there is the colour red, this indicates disease of the muscles. This diagnosis is confirmed if the person craves salt flavour.

If there is the colour yellow, this indicates disease of the nose and throat. This diagnosis is confirmed if the person craves sweet flavour.

If there is the colour black, this indicates disease of the bones. This diagnosis is confirmed if the person craves sour flavour.

If there is the colour white, this indicates disease of the skin. This diagnosis is confirmed if the person craves pungent flavour.

If there is the colour green, this indicates disease of the nervous system. This diagnosis is confirmed if the person craves bitter flavour.

7
Acupuncture and Moxa

Preparing for Acupuncture

Those who wish to practise acupuncture should mediate frequently in silence. They should be honest and generous: in word and action. They should know the difference between beauty and ugliness.

— *Book 8.1*

For acupuncture to be effective in healing the body, one must first heal the spirit.

— *Book 8.1*

Purpose of Treatment

The purpose of acupuncture is to supply what is lacking, and to drain off excess. When the needle is applied to places which are hollow and empty, these places will be replenished. When the needle is applied to places which are full and solid, these places will be drained.

— *Book 8.1*

HUANG DI

Principles of Treatment

Those who are experts in acupuncture follow the principle of Yin to draw out Yang; and they follow the principle of Yang to draw out Yin. They use the right hand to treat illnesses on the left side; and they use the left hand to treat illnesses on the right side.

— *Book 8.1*

When the pulse is beating strongly, the healer should apply cauterisation by burning moxa in the area of Yin, and needles of acupuncture in the area of Yang. When the pulse is weak, the healer should apply the needles of acupuncture in the area of Yang, and cauterisation by burning moxa in the area of Yin.

— *Book 8.4*

Variety of Treatment

The wise healer is capable of applying every type of treatment: acupuncture with flint needles and with metal needles; herbal medicines; moxibustion; and massage. The healer should diagnose each patient, and then apply the appropriate combination of these treatments.

— *Book 4.1*

ACUPUNCTURE AND MOXA

When a person's body is balanced and content, but the mind and emotions are in distress, cure the distress by using both moxa treatment and acupuncture.

When a person's body is balanced and content, when the emotions are tranquil, but when the mind is in distress, use acupuncture only.

When a person's body is balanced and content, when the mind is tranquil, but when the emotions are in distress, use moxa and breathing exercises.

When a person's body is ill, and when the mind and emotions are in distress, use acupuncture, moxa, breathing exercises and herbal medicine. — *Book 7.4*

Applying Acupuncture

To apply acupuncture without understanding the three regions of the body and the twelve sub-divisions is to commit a grave error. The vital substances of the body will be scattered and spoiled, and evil influences will reign within the body.

— *Book 6.3*

The human being has four main arteries and twelve subsidiary vessels. The four main arteries correspond to the four seasons, and the twelve subsidiary vessels to the twelve months. — *Book 2.3*

The human being has three hundred and sixty-five small ducts. These protect the life-force, and prevent evil influences from entering. When acupuncture is applied correctly to these ducts, it causes evil influence to depart.

— *Book 3.3*

When a person has an ulcer, the healer should pierce the area of the Yin region of the foot. If this does not bring a cure, the healer should pierce three times the palm of the hand in the area of the Yin region, and also pierce the arteries and veins between the shoulder and the back.

When the stomach of a person is excessively full, and cannot be pressed down with the hand, the healer should pierce the hand in the area of Yang.

When a person is suffering from cholera, the healer should pierce the Yin region which is three inches beside the backbone. There should be five piercings, using the round end of the needle.

When a person is suffering fits of anxiety, the healer should pierce each hand five times in the Yin area of the foot. The healer should also pierce three times the Yin area which is five inches above the ankle.

— *Book 8.4*

Using the Needle

The needle should be inserted when the patient is inhaling. The needle should be left for a while, and the patient should breathe quietly. The needle should be turned a little when the patient is inhaling. The needle should be take out when the patient is exhaling; it should be withdrawn slowly, and only come out completely when the patient has completely exhaled.

– *Book 8.3*

When acupuncture does not cure a disease immediately, it should be repeated. The needle should be applied quietly and with the utmost care.

– *Book 4.5*

8
Passion and Restraint

Benefits of Sex

A person should not abstain from sexual intercourse. Heaven must penetrate Earth; and Earth must be open to Heaven. Yin and Yang depend on one another, and develop from one another. The spirit of a person who abstains from sexual intercourse becomes stunted. Through the blending of a man's and a woman's vital essences in sexual union, both are enhanced and strengthened. But sexual activity must be controlled and guided, or else it becomes dangerous. — *Book 1*

Sexual intercourse, if conducted correctly, can bring seven benefits. The first is to concentrate the man's and the woman's vital essences. The second is to relax their minds and bodies. The third is to strength their internal organs. The fourth is to stimulate their blood circulation. The fifth is to strengthen their muscles, through the exertion involved. The sixth is to strengthen their bones. The seventh is to bring greater harmony of the emotions. — *Book 16*

Sexual Unity

People may suffer great weakness and debility because they do not conduct sexual intercourse correctly. Those who are expert in sexual intercourse are like good cooks who know how to blend the five flavours into a tasty broth. The perfect sexual union of man and woman is like the union of Heaven and Earth; in sexual intercourse a man and a woman may experience perfect harmony of Yang and Yin.

— *Book 1*

Prior to sexual union the man and the woman must harmonise their moods. They should sit close to one another, with the woman on the man's right. He may press her waist and caress her body, whispering words of love in her ear. Then, when they are both ready, they may kiss, the man sucking the woman's lower lip, and the woman sucking the man's upper lip. They may then feed on each other's saliva. Through caressing and kissing a thousand charms will unfold, and a hundred sorrows will be forgotten.

But if, as they seek to harmonise their moods, it becomes clear that one of them is not happy and cannot be aroused, then they should desist.

— *Book 4*

Sexual Desire

Just as there are five internal organs, there are five sexual desires. When the man and the woman start to breathe deeply and swallow their saliva, their lung desire is roused. When they whisper words of love to one another, their heart desire is roused. When they clasp one another in their arms, their pancreas desire is aroused. When their sexual organs become filled with blood, their liver desire is roused. When their sexual organs become moist, their kidney desire is roused.

— *Book 11*

Sexual Technique (1)

If the man moves and the woman does not respond, or if the woman is roused and the man does not comply, then the sexual act will both injure the man and harm the woman. This is because it will cause disunity and imbalance between Yin and Yang. Only if there is true unity of desire, and thence unity of movement, will the man and woman derive pleasure and benefit.

— *Book 3*

Sexual Technique (2)

Deep and shallow, slow and quick, straight and slanting thrusts – intercourse should involve a variety of movements, each with its own characteristics. A slow thrust should resemble the movement of a carp on a hook. A quick thrust should resemble a flight of birds against the wind. Inserting and withdrawing, moving up and down, moving from left to right and right to left, changing from deep to shallow and from shallow to deep, changing from slow to quick and from quick to slow – all these different movements should be correlated with great care. One must apply each movement at the proper time, and not cling to one style alone to serve one's immediate pleasure. *– Book 4*

Sexual Technique (3)

There are nine positions for sexual intercourse. The first is called the Turning Dragon; the second, the Tiger's Thread; the third, the Monkey's Attack; the fourth, the Cleaving Cicada; the fifth, the Mounting Turtle; the sixth, the Fluttering Phoenix Bird; the seventh, the Rabbit Sucking its Hair; the eighth, Overlapping Fish Scales; the ninth, Cranes with Joined Necks.

– Book 12

Restraining Emission

Some men believe that the pleasure of the sexual act lies in ejaculation. But after ejaculation the man's body is tired, his ears are buzzing, his eyes are heavy with sleep, his throat is parched, and his limbs inert. Although he has experience a brief moment of joy, the pleasure does not last. Yet if the man has sexual intercourse without ejaculating, his vital essence is strengthened, his body remains energetic, and his hearing and vision are acute. Moreover, although he has restrained his passion his love for the woman will increase.

— *Book 18*

The man's semen is his vital Yang essence. In Spring a man can allow himself to ejaculate once every three days; in Summer and Autumn twice a month. During the winter he should save up his semen, and not ejaculate at all. In this way he uses the winter to store up Yang.

— *Book 19*

When during the sexual act the man feels he is about to ejaculate, but wishes to restrain himself, he must firmly press with the fore and middle finger of the left hand a spot between the scrotum and the anus. At the same time he must inhale deeply, without holding his breath, and gnash his teeth. Then the semen will be activated, but not emitted. The activated semen will go to the brain, and enhance his mental faculties.

— *Book 18*

A man aged 15 can emit semen as often as once or twice a day, depending on his strength. A man aged 30 can emit semen once every one or two days, depending on his strength. A man aged 40 may emit semen once every three or four days, depending on his strength. A man aged 50 may emit semen once every five or ten days, depending on his strength. A man aged 60 may emit semen once every ten or twenty days, depending on his strength. A man aged 70 may emit semen once a month if he is strong; if he is weak, he should no longer emit semen.

Bibliography

HUANG DI, *Nei Ching Su Wien* (*The Yellow Emperor's Classic of Internal Medicine*) trans. Ilza Veith, University of California Press, Los Angeles, 1966.

VAN GULIK, R. H., *Sexual Life in Ancient China*, E. J. Brill [Leiden], 1974.

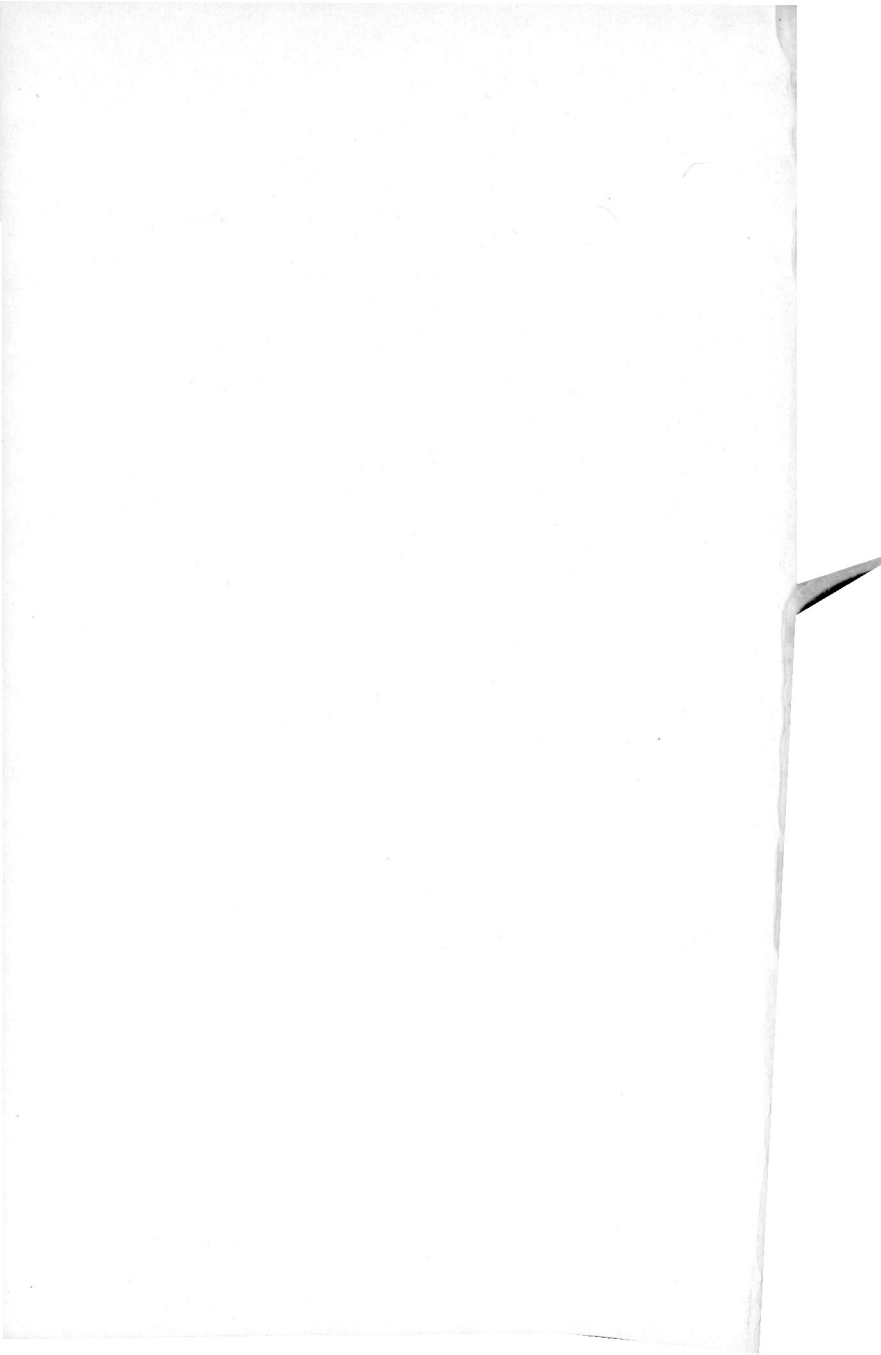